Lavender

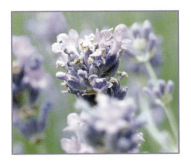

Jessie Hawkins

SILVERLEAF
PRESS

Silverleaf Press Books are available exclusively
through Independent Publishers Group.

For details write or telephone
Independent Publishers Group, 814 North Franklin St.
Chicago, IL 60610, (312) 337-0747

Silverleaf Press
8160 South Highland Drive
Sandy, Utah 84093

ISBN-13:978-1933317-78-6

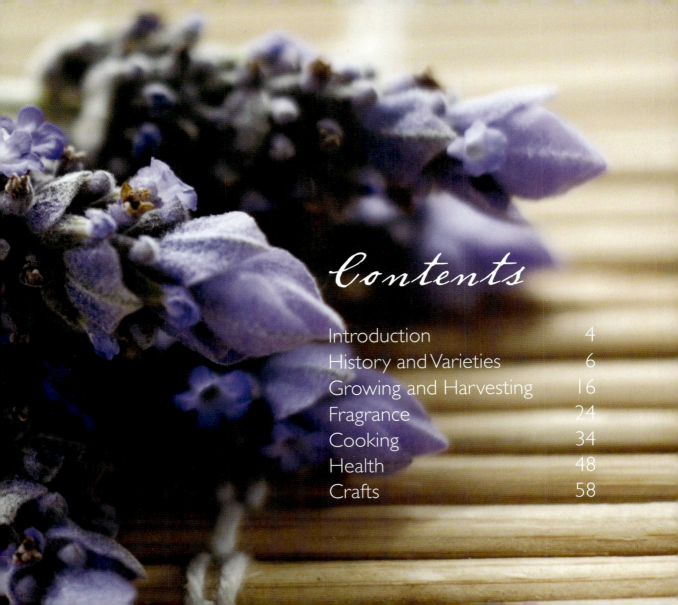

Contents

Introduction

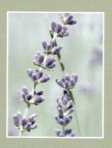

Lavender—just the name conjures thoughts of romantic, faraway Victorian chaise lounges or famed Roman baths. After all, it is the herb reputed to have helped Cleopatra sway Mark Anthony to her side (though her unmatched beauty did seem to play a part). I doubt there is an herb with the history and legend that lavender does. This simple Mediterranean herb has made its way across the world, captivating cultures throughout history.

Now, years away from public baths and tussie mussies, lavender is still an integral part of our culture. Just as in civilizations past, lavender is a staple among bath luxuries and our headaches can still be soothed by a temple rub made with its precious oil. It graces fine tables worldwide and lends its sweet scent to candles, salts, and bowls of potpourri in homes across the world.

Join me as we explore the many uses for this herb, from growing and harvesting to crafting, medicine, and even baking. I am sure you will be as awed as I am once you discover the many uses of this seemingly simple yet classic herb.

Jessie Hawkins, MH

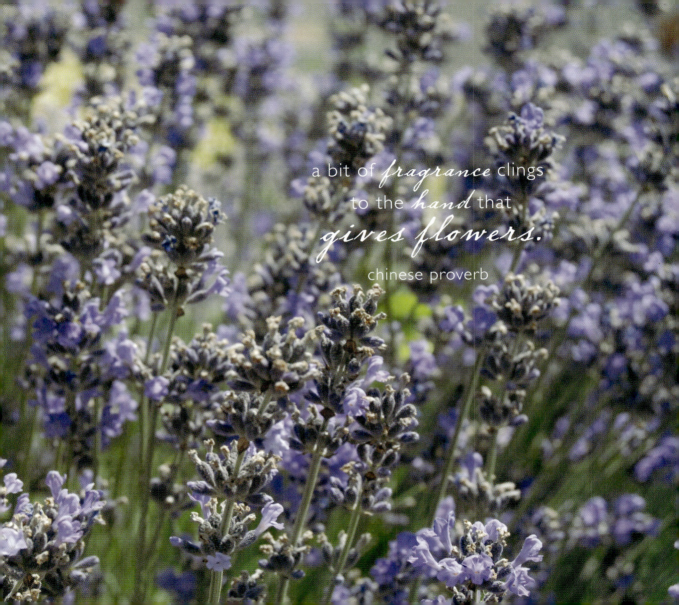

a bit of *fragrance* clings
to the *hand* that
gives flowers.

chinese proverb

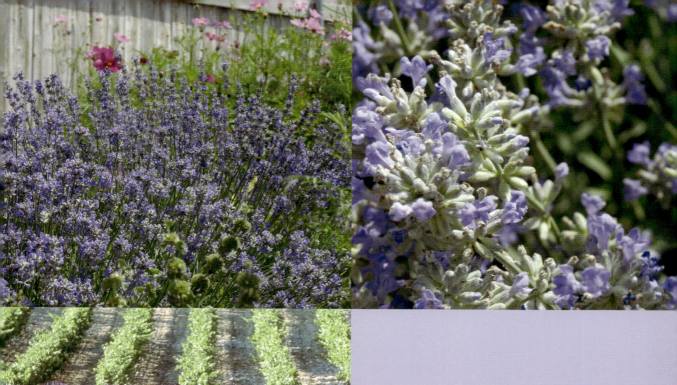

one faces the *future*
with one's *past.*

pearl s. buck

History and Varieties

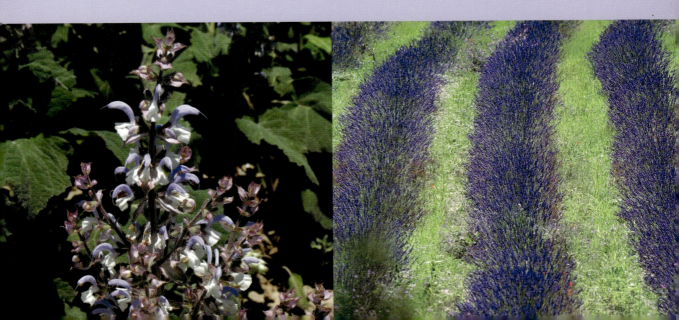

History

Lavender Names

The name "lavender" comes from the Latin root word "lavare," which means "to wash." Throughout history, lavender has always been associated with the bath. From the earliest Roman bathhouses to our modern lavender vanilla concoctions, lavender has been the herb of choice for bathing. In medieval and renaissance Europe, the washing women were often called "lavenders" because they were followed by the famous lavender scent. They would use lavender to fragrance clothing by drying it out on bushes of lavender to absorb the scent. Monks also grew lavender during this time, along with other medicinal herbs.

Egyptian Mummies

The first use we know of lavender, which is native to the Mediterranean, is slightly less romantic then what this herb has a reputation for now. The ancient Egyptian mummies often contained lavender, which was used heavily during the preservation process. In addition to the fragrance it offered, lavender also provided antibacterial properties useful in preservation.

Roman Baths

Roman bathhouses offered a dramatic change of pace for this fragrant herb. Lavender was the herb of choice in public bathhouses

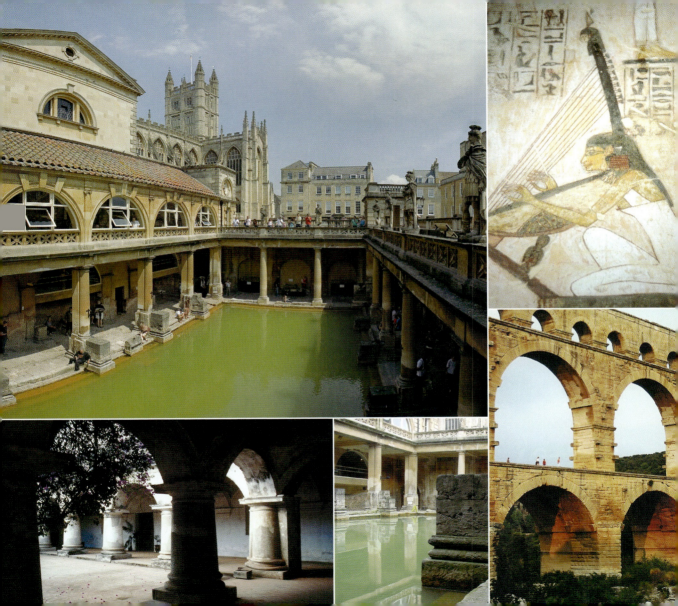

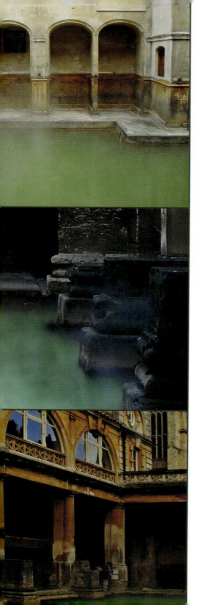

and had a wide reputation for refreshing the skin. Again, the fragrance and the antibacterial properties of this herb make it an excellent choice. The going rate for lavender flowers during this time was 100 denarii a pound, which was roughly a month's salary for an average person. Upon leaving the bathhouses, men would often apply a touch of lavender for its clean refreshing scent. Cleopatra also reportedly used this scent in seducing Julius Caesar and Mark Anthony.

Simple Lavender Bath

A famed Roman bath is easy to replicate in your own home. Simply sprinkle ¼ cup lavender petals over a warm bath and let them steep 5–10 minutes. For easy removal, petals can be placed in a muslin tea bag before adding to the bath.

Medieval and Renaissance Europe

Lavender's romantic reputation continued during the renaissance period, in which it was commonly used as a laundry fragrance. Sprigs of lavender would be placed between linens to keep them smelling fresh, and the plant itself became a stylish decoration as hedging in gardens and as an ornamental plant. It was the Victorians, though, who brought the plant indoors. They also began to widely use the herb for sachets and the classic lavender wands.

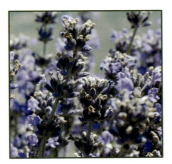

Lavender Wands

13 sprigs of fresh lavender
2 yards (1.8m) of satin ribbon (½ or ¾-inch (1–2cm) thick)

1. Arrange the lavender stalks so that the flowers are all at the same end, and tie them together with the ribbon, leaving one end longer than the other.
2. Taking the long end of the ribbon, weave it through the lavender flowers as you would a basket.
3. When you reach the top, continue back down the wand, making new rows in between the old rows.
4. Finish with a bow at the base of the flowers.

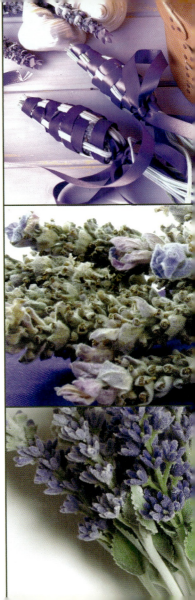

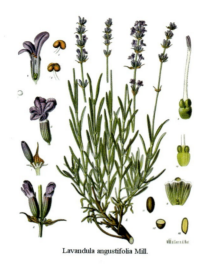

Lavandula angustifolia Mill.

Varieties

There exist 28 varieties of lavender, and many more offshoots. The most common ones are listed here, but the names are often used loosely and many times one variety is termed another due to the similarity of the flowers.

English

English lavender is the queen of all lavenders. Usually *Lavandula angustifolia*, but also including *Lavandula officinalis*, *Lavandula vera*, *Lavandula delphinensis* and *Lavandula spica*, this group of flowers is prized worldwide for its pure scent and culinary wonders. The flowers do not produce as much oil as other types, but the quality is far superior. The bright blue flowers and buds are dried for their decorative uses, and the fragrant oil has many uses in the kitchen and beyond.

French

French lavender (*Lavandula dentata*) is very different in both look and fragrance. The flowers are shaped differently and grow only a few petals between the buds. The buds and petals are slightly grayish looking, as opposed to the bright blueish purple we associate with the plant. This lavender is not grown as a culinary lavender, and it does not offer the sweet, floral scent of other lavenders used for essential oils.

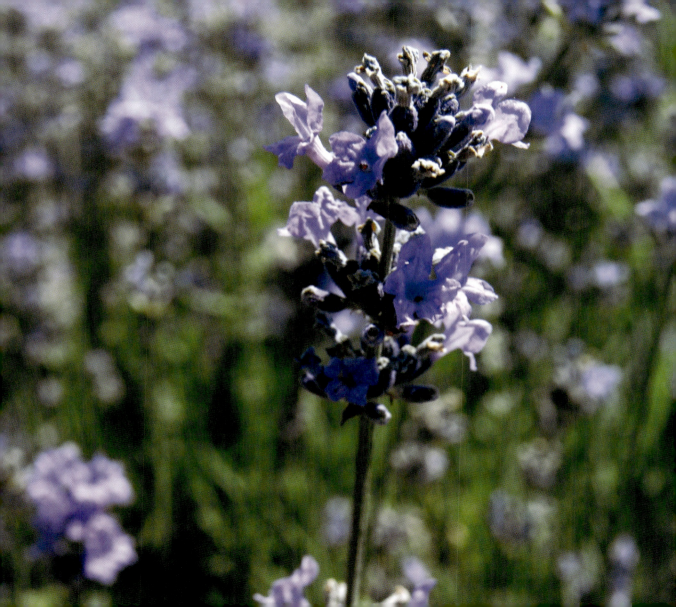

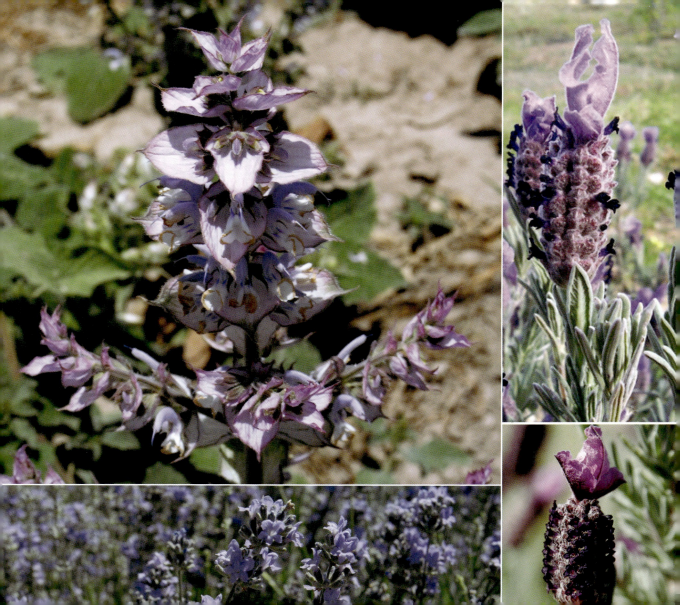

Spanish

Spanish lavender, Spike lavender, and Portuguese lavender are all known as *Lavandula latifolia*. This flower grows petals at the top of the flowering buds. Similar to French lavender, these flowers are not used for culinary purposes, and the fragrance is somewhat "medicinal" to many.

Bulgarian

Bulgarian lavender (which is actually *Lavandula angustifolia*, grown in Bulgaria) is perhaps the most commonly used for essential oil distillation. Not only does it offer a pure scent, but it is very affordable. As opposed to many other varieties of lavender essential oil, the oil Bulgarian lavender produces is much more true to dried lavender and has a very mellow and floral scent. Many report other lavenders as having a somewhat medicinal or camphoric scent to them. Try Bulgarian lavender essential oil in body care and room fragrances.

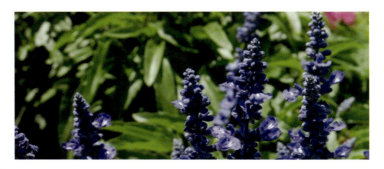

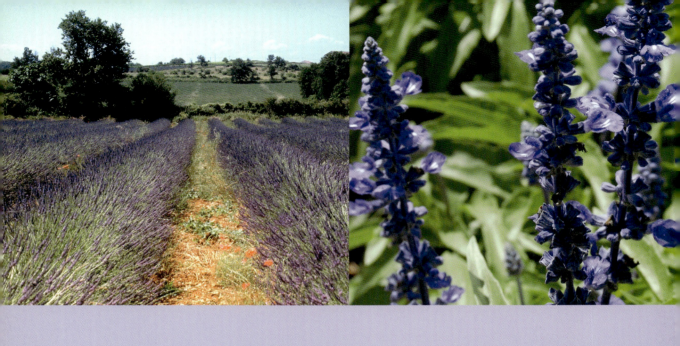

Growing and Harvesting

i hope that while so many
people are out *smelling*
the *flowers,* someone
is taking the time to
plant some.

herbert rappaport

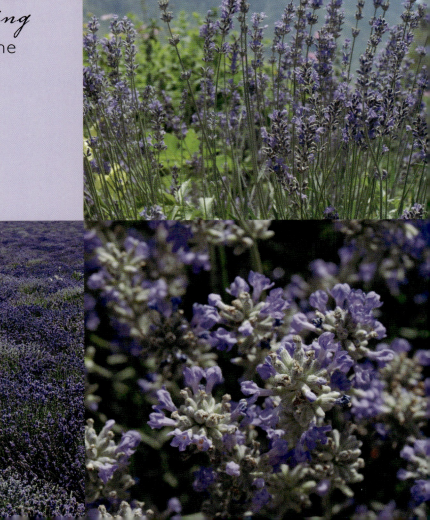

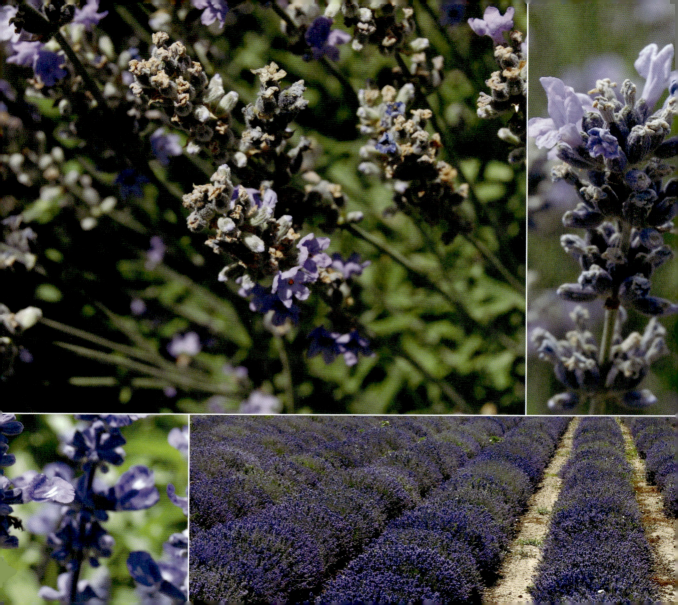

Basics

Lavenders consist of 28 plants in the mint family. This bushy shrub is a perennial favorite that grows quite well with other herbs such as hyssop and yarrow. The small purple flowers grow in a whorl pattern of 6–10 flowers forming spikes on 6–8-inch (15–20cm) stalks. The leaves are a silvery gray that grow in an opposite pattern up to 2 inches long. The entire shrub grows to an average of 2–3 feet (.5-1m) tall and puts forth its flowers in June and July.

Varieties

English lavender, or *Lavandula angustifolia*, is a good choice for growing in home gardens. Not only are they sweet smelling and beautiful, but they are also fairly easy to grow and dry well for crafts and decorative uses. Lavenders are slow to germinate, so buying well-established plants or seedlings is often your best bet.

Mediterranean Climate

Native to the Mountainous zones of the Mediterranean, lavender enjoys a hot, dry climate. In the US, we can expect optimal performance in zones 5–8 with a soil pH of 7 to 7.5. Outside of those zones, lavender can be grown in a container indoors. To recreate its native environment, use light soil with very good drainage, and be sure the plant gets full sun exposure. This desert plant will sometimes struggle in humid climates, but with some care it can easily be done. Try a raised bed for increased drainage, and be sure not to overwater. Or, for simplicity, you can grow lavendin, a hybrid of lavender that is more tolerant to humidity.

Landscaping

In addition to its beauty in the picturesque fields of lavender that grow purple blossoms as far as the eye can see, lavender can be admired as a wonderful addition to a professional home landscape. Its size is perfect as edging for walks, ponds, or gardens. Be sure to space the plants 12–15 inches (30–40cm) apart, and keep in mind the special growing requirements of lavender.

Containers

In difficult climates, container growing may be the best bet. Look for a container that is fairly large. Their root systems are pretty big for their size, though they do grow well in tight spaces. A rule of thumb is to keep the pot 1–2 inches (3–5cm) larger than the root ball. Be sure it has great drainage to reproduce the native climate, and if needed, drill some drainage holes of your own. As an extra measure, add gravel or sand to the bottom of the pot to ensure good drainage. With loose soil, and a location that offers 8 hours a day of sunlight, your lavender should do quite well. It will require more water than an outdoor plant, but not enough to water every day. Rather, wait until the soil is dry to water.

Cutting

The best time to cut most herbs is midmorning, after the dew has dried, but before the heat sets in. Look for the bottom third of the spike to blossom. When this happens, the lavender is ready to be cut. Be sure to use clean, sharp scissors, and cut the lavender stalks towards the bottom of the stem in bundles.

After the flowering season, prune the stems back about two thirds of the way. This will help boost your production and prevent the plant from becoming too woody.

Drying

Fresh lavender will retain its look and shape for up to a week in a vase with fresh water. To preserve the beauty and fragrance longer, consider drying the trimmings. To dry the plant, group the cuttings in bunches of 8–10 stalks. Tie together with a ribbon or raffia and hang upside down in a dark, dry room (such as a closet). Wait a few weeks, and be sure the stalks are totally dry before removing them. Once dried, they can be stored in larger bunches.

Dried Lavender Fire Logs

For an aromatic use of extra lavender, take a small bunch of the flowers and tie together as a mini log. Once the fire is going well, toss in a lavender log. Not only do they smell great, but the extra "logs" are a decorative touch to the fireplace hearth.

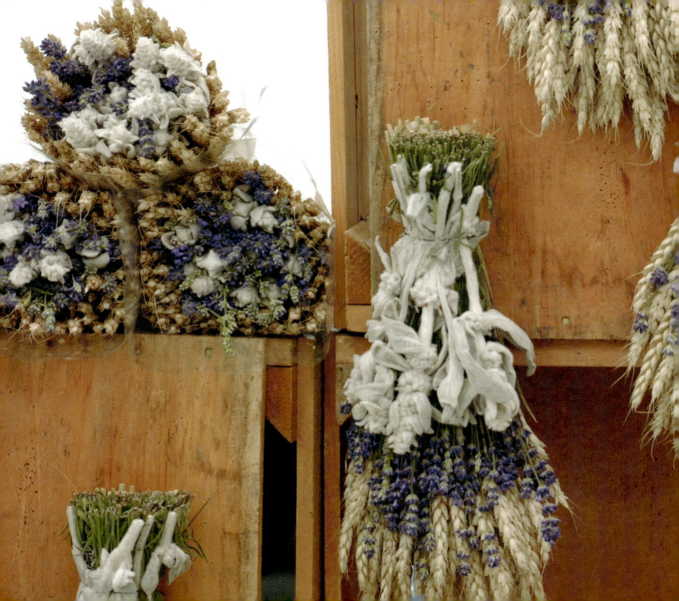

Storing

Once the lavender is fully dry, it is ready to be stored. First decide how to store it. This will depend on how you plan to use it. For mostly decorative and crafting purposes, you may want to keep the whole stalk. For potpourri or cooking, you only need the buds. If your plans are strictly culinary, you could even consider grinding the buds and storing the powder.

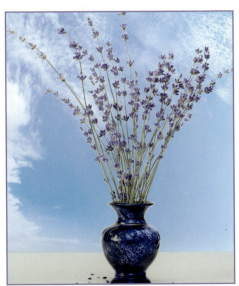

smell is a potent wizard that *transports* you across thousand of miles and all the *years* you have lived.

helen keller

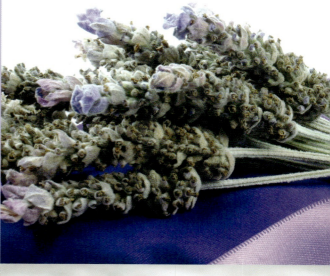

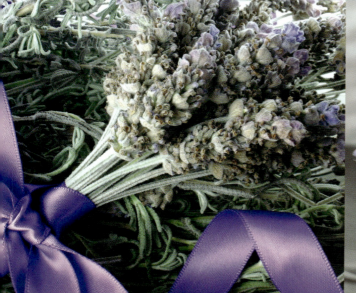

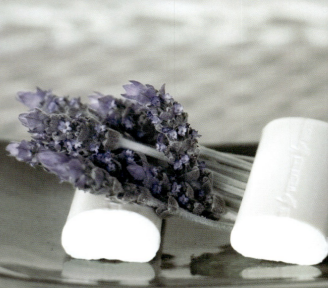

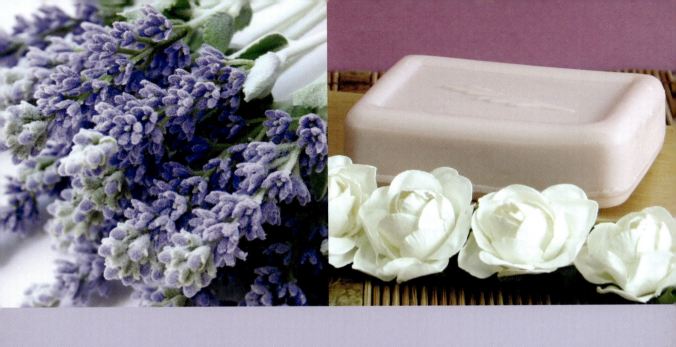

Fragrance

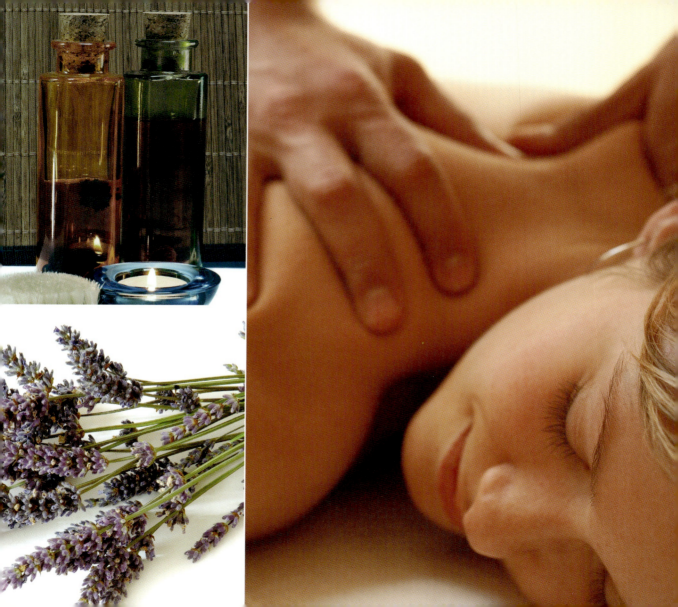

Essential Oil

An essential oil, also referred to as a volatile oil, is the oil obtained from certain parts of select herbs and plants. Lavender essential oil, commonly called lavender oil, is obtained from lavender flowers. Essential oils can be purchased from your local health food store or through several online retailers.

While essential oil cannot be made at home without expensive equipment, an infusion of lavender can be made simply with dried lavender plants. This infusion can be substituted for a diluted essential oil in any project.

Lavender Infusion

1 glass bottle
dried lavender buds
oil or vinegar

Fill the bottle with the lavender flowers and be sure to pack it tightly. Add the oil or vinegar slowly, and fill to ½ inch (1-2 cm) above the flowers. Let sit for 3 weeks, then strain the flowers out.

Aromatherapy

Aromatherapy is the art and science of using plant oils to enhance health and well-being. Aromatherapy literally means "to treat using scents." Plant oils have been used throughout history in Egypt, Italy, India, and China, but the term was first used by a French chemist named Rene-Maurice Gattefosse in 1937. Lavender oil is one of the most widely used and familiar aromatherapy oils. Only a pure lavender oil will work for aromatherapy purposes; artificial or synthetic scents are not chemically structured exactly the same. Lavender essential oil can be made from all species of the plant, but the most commonly used varieties are Spike lavender (*Lavandula latifolia*) and English lavender (*Lavandula angustifolia*).

Diffusing Lavender

Diffused lavender creates a calming and soothing effect. There are many ways to diffuse oils, but these are my favorite:

Water Diffusing

Bring 1 cup of water almost to the boiling point, then pour into a shallow bowl. Add 10 drops lavender oil to the water. The steam will cause the oils to diffuse into the room. This method will quickly diffuse the oil, but it will not last more than a few hours.

Reed Diffusing

Place 5–7 diffusing reeds into a glass bottle. Fill the bottle ⅔ with distilled water and 10–15 drops lavender oil. Turn the reeds upside down every 2–3 days to refresh the scent. This will diffuse the oil slower than the water method, and last longer. Every 7–9 days, change the water and reeds.

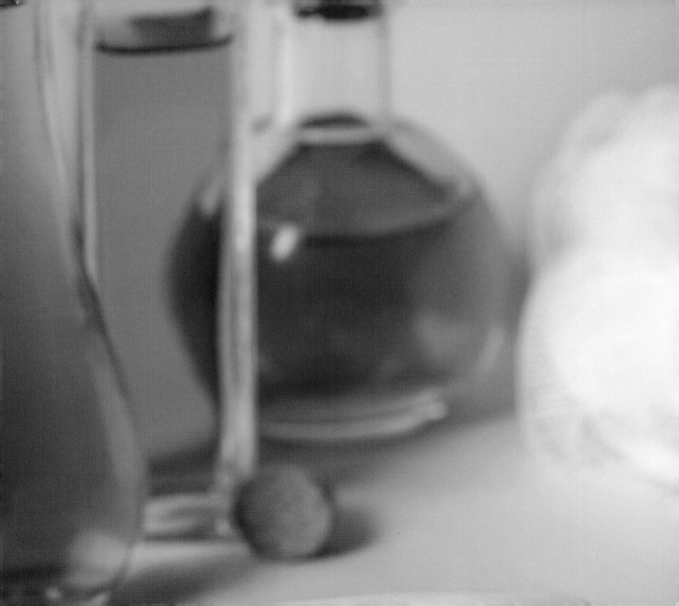

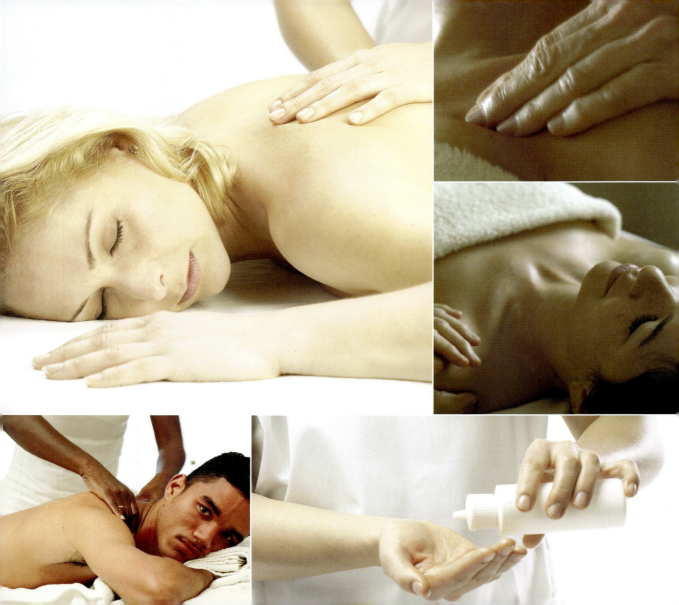

Using Lavender

Lavender Massage Oil

Nothing says massage quite like lavender. This traditional calming scent is the number one choice for relaxing after a long day. Making a massage oil is actually quite easy.

8 ounce glass bottle
3 ounces pure olive oil
3 ounces avocado oil
2 ounces grapeseed oil
25 drops lavender oil

Pour the oils into the bottle and cap. Shake very well to blend the oils thoroughly. To make a massage oil for children or babies, only use 10–15 drops of lavender.

Lavender Water

Lavender water is another way to infuse the scent into a room or car. It is also great as a natural body fragrance or linen spray. Lavender water can be purchased, or you can make your own.

2 cups distilled water
½ cup grain alcohol (vodka works well)
30 drops lavender essential oil

Pour the water, alcohol, and oil into a clean, sterile bottle and cap with a spritzing top. This blend will last 10–12 months. Warning: It is flammable.

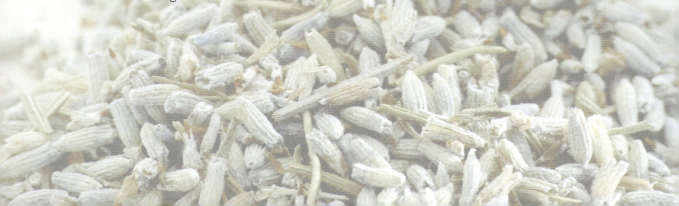

Dried Lavender

Dried lavender makes a beautiful decoration. And as the lavender oil is still in the buds, it drifts into the room, offering its enticing scent. Dried lavender can be bought by the scoopful, which is common for the flowers. If you are lucky, you can also find dried lavender stalks.

Dried lavender flowers are best displayed by themselves for optimal lavender essence. Place ½ cup to 1 cupful of the buds into a shallow decorative bowl. These can be placed throughout the house. Smaller rooms, such as powder rooms, will hold a more concentrated scent.
Lavender stalks can be bundled together for a centerpiece or mantle decoration. Simply tie together a handful of dried lavender stalks with raffia or a satin ribbon. Be sure the tallest stalks are in the center and the ends are cut to the same level. Stand the stalks upright in the room of your choice.

Lavender Potpourris

Lavender blends well with other scents, making it a desirable anchor for a potpourri blend.
Try the light citrus blend in a kitchen or breakfast room and the deeper, more floral blend in a bedroom or living room.

Lavender Orange Blend

2 cups lavender flowers
1 cup orange peel
½ cup lemon peel
¼ cup juniper berries
¼ cup cloves
¼ cup marigold flowers

Deep Lavender Floral Blend

2 cups lavender flowers
1 cup rose petals
½ cup jasmine
¼ cup rosemary
¼ cup bay leaves

Lavender Linen Powder

Legend has it that couples that sleep with lavender in their linens never quarrel. True to the legend or not, the captivating fragrance makes it well worth the try!

1 cup baking soda
½ cup cornstarch or arrowroot powder
½ cup white clay (kaolin clay)
15–25 drops lavender essential oil

In a medium bowl mix together the powders. Slowly pour the oil in and stir until well combined with no clumps. Store in a covered jar by the bed and dust fresh linens generously.

Lavender

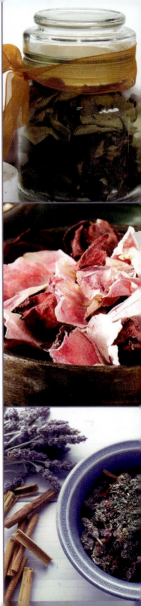

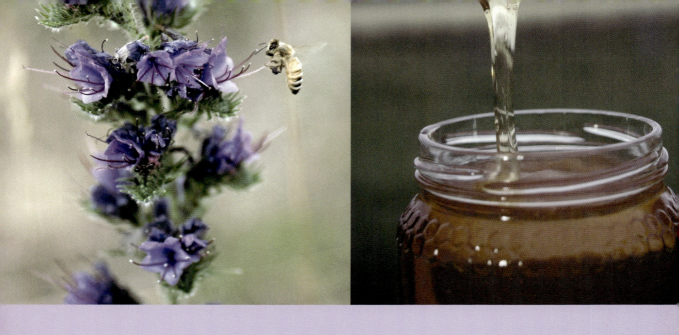

Cooking

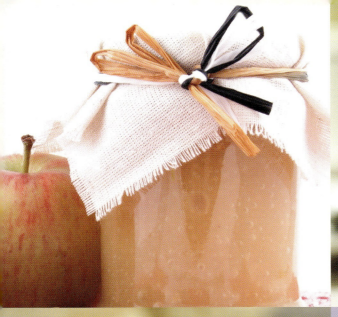

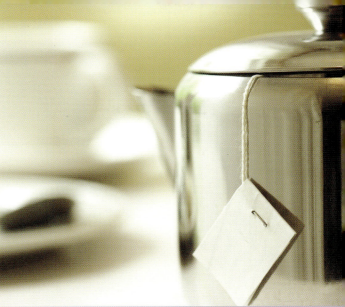

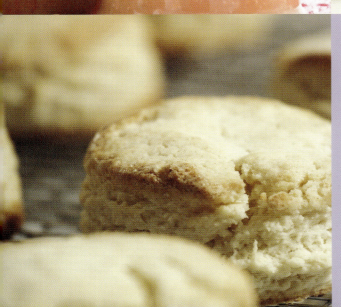

you don't have to *cook*
fancy or complicated
masterpieces—just
good food from *fresh*
ingredients.

julia child

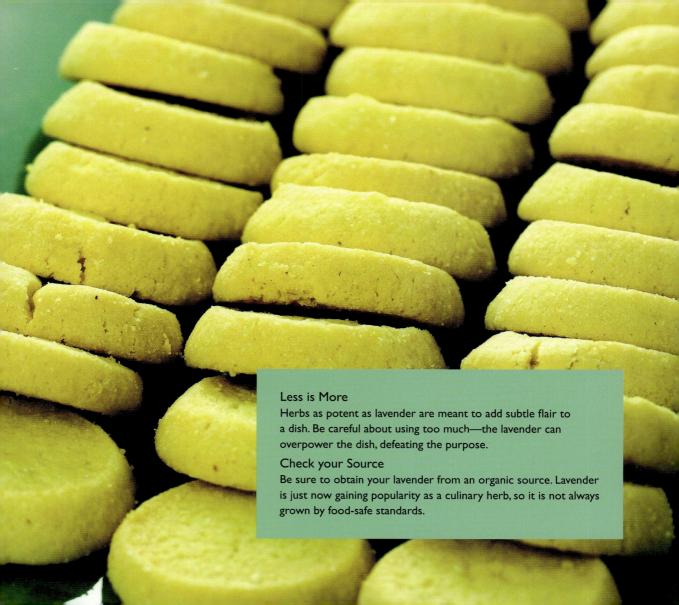

Less is More
Herbs as potent as lavender are meant to add subtle flair to
a dish. Be careful about using too much—the lavender can
overpower the dish, defeating the purpose.

Check your Source
Be sure to obtain your lavender from an organic source. Lavender
is just now gaining popularity as a culinary herb, so it is not always
grown by food-safe standards.

Cooking

Edible flowers are quickly gaining respect in the culinary world. Lavender, a member of the mint family and Mediterranean native, is a prime example of the unique flavor and presentation that flowering herbs can impart to a dish. Most Mediterranean herbs blend well together and can be added to most meats and vegetables effortlessly. Try composing your own *Herbs de Provence* blend with lavender, oregano, rosemary, thyme, and sage, or try out one of our recipes to introduce your taste buds to this delightful herb.

Lavender Lemon Cookies

1 teaspoon lemon zest
¼ cup organic lavender buds
1 cup organic sugar
1 cup butter, room temperature
1 egg
juice from 1 fresh lemon
2 cups all-purpose flour
¼ teaspoon baking soda
¼ teaspoon baking powder

Mix lemon zest with ¼ cup lavender buds. Set aside. In a mixer with the paddle attachment, beat sugar and butter until creamy, about 1 minute. Add the egg and lemon juice. Mix well. Sift together flour, baking soda, and baking powder. Slowly add to the butter mixture. When well incorporated, form into a ball and chill overnight. Form the dough into 1-inch balls and dip the tops into the lavender lemon mixture. Bake at 350°F (177°C) for 10–12 minutes.

Biscuits with Lavender Honey

Lavender honey is made by bees that only gather from lavender flowers. Most good lavender honey comes from France and can be purchased through specialty shops.

1 teaspoon warm water
1 tablespoon honey
1 package active dry yeast
1 ½ cups all-purpose flour
1 cup white wheat flour (as opposed to red wheat—can be found in health food stores or specialty grocery stores)
2 teaspoons baking powder
½ teaspoon salt
½ teaspoon baking soda
1 stick cold unsalted butter, cut into small pieces
1 cup buttermilk
1 cup lavender honey

Dissolve honey in warm water. Add yeast and let sit 4–5 minutes. Sift together the flours, baking powder, salt, and baking soda. Add the butter, and cut it in until the mixture is coarse and the butter is well blended. Add the buttermilk and yeast and stir to mix.

When the mixture becomes a thick dough, place it onto a well-floured surface and knead to be sure all is mixed well. Roll out the dough to about a half-inch (1–2 cm) thick. Cut biscuits with a 2-inch (5cm) cutter. Let rise 30–45 minutes then bake in a 400°F oven for 8–10 minutes. Serve with lavender honey and butter.

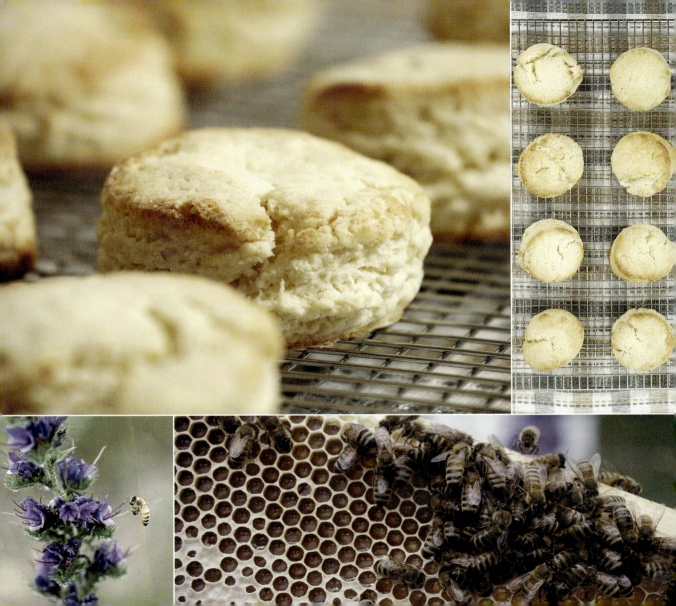

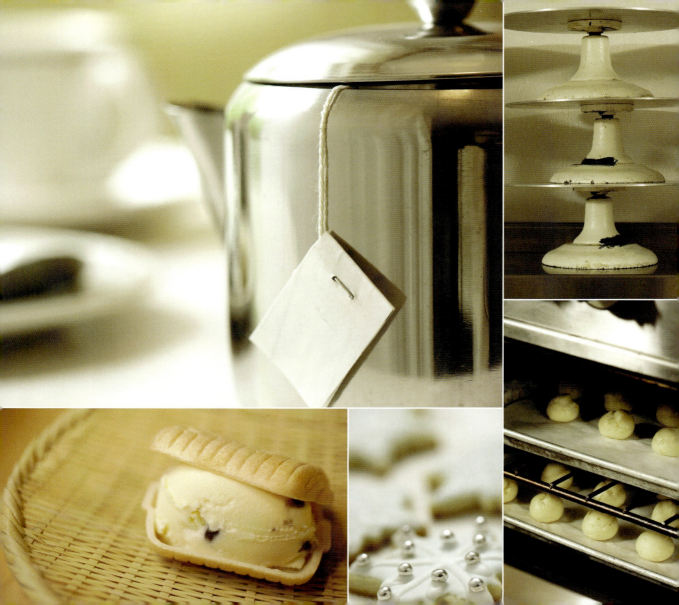

Lavender Tea Cakes

½ cup chilled butter
I cup organic sugar
I egg
I tablespoon milk
I teaspoon lemon essential oil or vanilla extract
2 cups white wheat flour
½ teaspoon baking powder
¼ teaspoon salt
¼ cup crushed lavender buds
2 tablespoons lavender buds (for decoration)

Cut butter into sugar. Add the egg, milk, and flavoring. Mix well. Add dry ingredients and mix until no lumps remain. *For shapes:* Put in the fridge overnight. Remove and roll out to ½-inch (1–2 cm) and cut into shapes. Butter and flour a cookie sheet and place shapes onto sheet. Bake at 350°F (177°C) for 6–8 minutes. Top warm cakes with whole lavender buds. *For freeform cakes:* Scoop into 1 tablespoon mounds onto prepared cookie sheet. Bake at 350°F (177°C) for 6–8 minutes. Top warm cakes with whole lavender buds. Cakes should be a light golden brown. Serve with lavender honey.

Apple Jelly with Lavender Sprigs

3 pounds apples (1.4kg)
2–3 cups water
3 cups sugar
dried organic lavender sprigs

Wash, peel, and core the apples. Cut them into 1-inch (2.5 cm) cubes. Place apples into a large pot and cover with water. Bring water to a boil, then lower heat to simmer apples. Cook until apples are soft throughout (about 20 minutes). Strain the mixture with a fine mesh strainer.

Add the sugar and bring back to a boil for only 8–10 minutes. Test the mixture for a gel by adding a small amount to a bowl of cool water.

When it is thickened, remove from heat and ladle into jars. Before sealing, add 2–3 lavender sprigs to each jar, then cap and seal.

Chicken with Herbs de Provence

2 tablespoons dried lavender
2 tablespoons dried thyme
1 tablespoon dried oregano
1 teaspoon dried basil
1 teaspoon dried rosemary
½ teaspoon dried sage
½ teaspoon each salt and pepper

Blend herbs together. Set aside 2 tablespoons mixture for chicken. Store remaining herbs for later.

2 tablespoons butter, melted
2 tablespoons herb mixture
4 chicken breasts

Mix butter and herbs together. Pound the chicken to ½-inch (1–2 cm) thick. Grill over medium heat for 4–5 minutes on each side. Brush with butter mixture on each side. Serve warm with potatoes, grilled veggies, and focaccia bread.

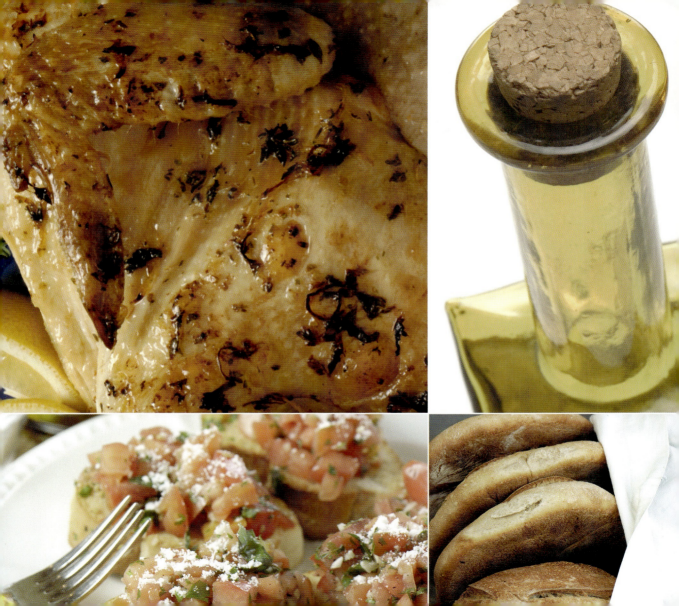

Lavender Focaccia

2 packages active dry yeast
1 teaspoon honey
1 cup warm water
¾ cup water
¼ cup extra virgin olive oil, plus extra to drizzle on the bread
1 teaspoon salt
4½ to 5 cups unbleached flour
3 tablespoons lavender buds
2 tablespoons rosemary
coarse salt

Dissolve honey and yeast into the warm water. Let sit 5–10 minutes. Put the remaining water, oil, and salt into a mixer with a dough hook. Blend together with the yeast mixture, add the herbs and flour 1 cup at a time until a smooth dough forms. Knead 4–5 minutes. Let rise an hour or until doubled. Punch down. Divide into two parts and form into 2 dough rounds. Let rise again on an oiled baking sheet for 30–45 minutes. Sprinkle coarse salt over the top. Bake at 400°F (204°C) degrees for 15–20 minutes.

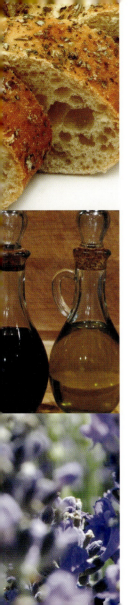

Lavender Bruschetta *(with cheeses, tomatoes, and lavender)*

1 baguette
3–4 ripe Roma tomatoes, diced
1 clove garlic, crushed
1 tablespoon lavender
2 teaspoons basil
coarse salt and pepper to taste
extra virgin olive oil
3 tablespoons grated Parmesan cheese

In a small bowl, toss the tomatoes, garlic, 1 tablespoon olive oil, lavender and basil together. Chill 4–5 hours to allow the flavors to mellow and blend. Slice the baguette into 1-inch slices, brush with olive oil, and bake until lightly toasted. Spoon 1–2 tablespoons mixture over each slice. Top with grated cheese and salt and pepper to taste and serve immediately.

Lavender Vinaigrette

1 teaspoon lavender buds
1 teaspoon basil
1 teaspoon Dijon mustard
3 tablespoons olive oil
2 tablespoons red wine vinegar

Mix the vinegar with the herbs and mustard until well blended. Whisk quickly, while slowly drizzling the oil into the mix. Continue mixing until well incorporated. Add salt and pepper to taste. Serve over a bed of Romaine with quartered Roma tomatoes, sliced cucumbers, and grated Parmesan cheese.

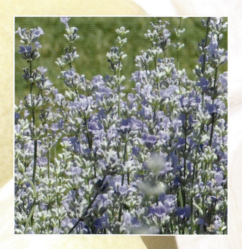

Lavender Limeade

1½ cups sugar
6 cups ice water
¼ cup lavender buds
2 cups ice
juice of 5 fresh limes
½ thinly sliced lime
1 lavender sprig

Bring water and sugar to a boil. Add lavender and steep for 10 minutes. Strain the lavender with a fine mesh strainer. Add the lime juice and ice. Stir well.

Add the sliced limes and lavender sprig. Enjoy!

Lavender

Lavender Lemon Sorbet

Nothing blends better with lavender's exotic Mediterranean flavor than tangy lemon. Try this tasty sorbet with lavender honey drizzled over the top instead of the traditional chocolate or caramel. Decorate with sprigs of fresh lavender for a culinary delight.

¾ cup organic sugar (also known as dried cane juice)
I cup hot water
zest of one lemon
3 tablespoons organic lavender buds
I cup fresh lemon juice
ice cream maker

In a medium pan, blend the cane juice with I cup hot water. Bring to a boil over high heat then reduce heat and simmer until it thickens and all the sugar is dissolved (about 4–6 minutes). Add the zest, buds, and juice, and set aside to cool about 5–10 minutes. Strain out the buds (if desired), and pour into an ice cream maker. Freeze according to the directions on the machine.

look to your *health;* and
if you have it, praise god and
value it next to conscience;
for health is the second
blessing that we mortals
are capable of, a blessing
money can't buy.

izaak walton

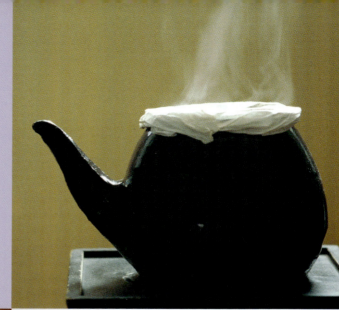

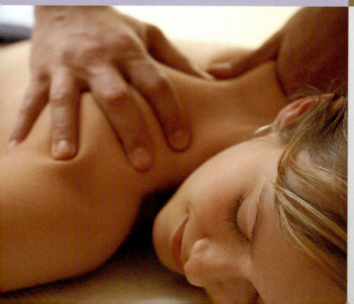

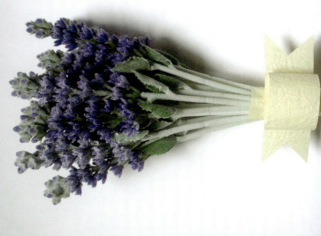

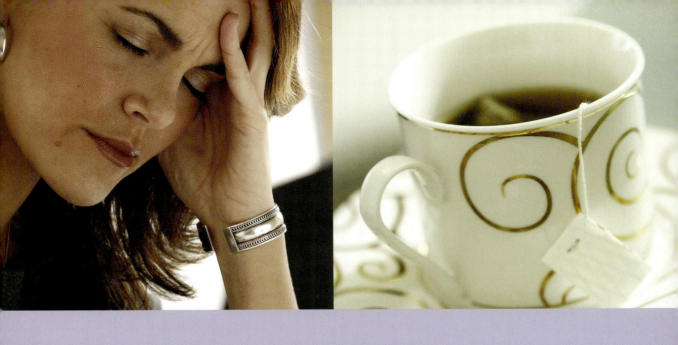

Health

Science and Uses

Lavender is one of the most well-known medicinal herbs. It enjoyed a long membership in the British Pharmacopia for over 200 years and is still approved by the German Commission E for various upsets. Lavender oil was used as a disinfectant for wounds until WWI. Scientifically, lavender has shown antiseptic properties, which validates the original uses of the herb.

Four Thieves

According to the legend, four thieves went around during the French plagues of the early 1700s robbing graves and taking items from the homes of plague victims. At first, the authorities disregarded the thieves, believing they would soon die from the plague. But time passed and they continued robbing and plundering, seemingly immune to the plague. Finally, authorities captured them and threatened to kill them unless they divulged their secret, "How did they avoid catching the plague?" They chose to disclose their secret and confessed that they came from a family of perfumers who had created an herbal vinegar that protected them from the disease. Lavender was a key component in this famous recipe, which was used until the late 1800s.

The following recipe varies from the original, but contains these common herbs and is simple to make at home:
Combine approximately 2 tablespoons of each: lavender, rosemary,

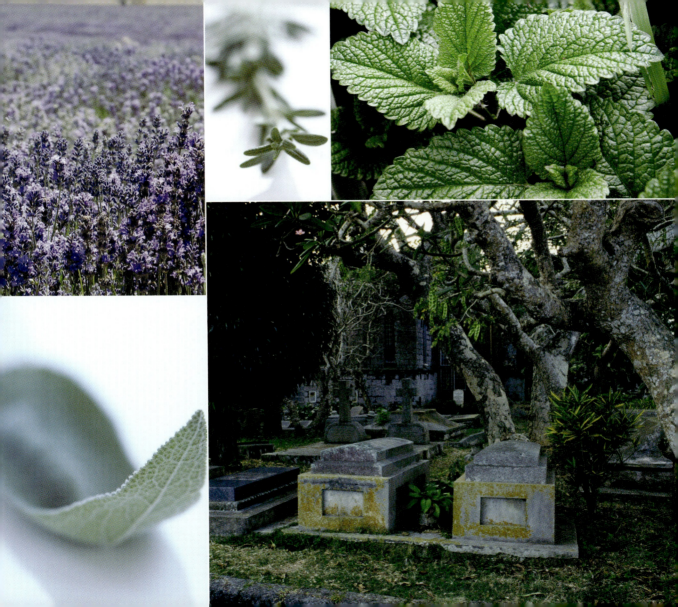

sage, rue, and mint in a canning jar, and cover with 2 cups apple cider vinegar. Leave for 4–8 weeks to steep. Strain and add 2 tablespoons chopped garlic. Steep for another week or two, then strain into another jar. "Four Thieves Vinegar" has been used in salad dressings, as a room spray, as an antiseptic wash, and even as a bug spray.

Temple Rub

Lavender is perhaps most widely known for its calming, soothing scent. This herb gives off a distinct fragrance that many report to be stress relieving. To take advantage of this simple benefit, make a temple rub. This balm can be rubbed into the temples for headaches, or it can help to compensate for over-stimulated children or a stressful day at the office.

2 tablespoons olive oil
½ teaspoon beeswax
25 drops Bulgarian lavender oil
½ ounce (14g) metal tin

In a glass measuring cup, melt the wax with the oil in the microwave (for roughly 25–30 seconds, depending on the microwave). Quickly stir in the lavender oil , and pour into the metal tin. Cap immediately and set aside to cool.

First Aid

Lavender is the main component for any herbal first aid kit. The essential oil is one of the very few that herbalists suggest can be used undiluted, or "neat," on the skin. It can be a powerful allergen, however, and is to be used with caution. (Do not use lavender if you have a history of allergies to the mint family, or are unsure of your allergies. And do not use neat on babies or young children.) In the absence of lavender oil, lavender tea can be used externally, though it is much less potent.

Lavender first aid uses generally cover the following:
Minor burns: * Lavender oil can be dropped directly on the minor burn (such as a sunburn) or mixed with aloe for combined relief.
Headaches: Lavender can be used as a temple rub (see page 52) or as a room freshener for headache relief.
Bites: Many insect bites can be relieved with lavender essential oil applied directly to the bite.
Sore muscles: Lavender essential oil can be diluted into a carrier oil (such as olive or grapeseed) and massaged into sore muscles to provide relief.
*Note: In the event of a major burn or wound, seek a physician's care.

Portable Lavender

The many health uses of lavender are often needed most when you are out and about. Headaches or sore muscles are frequently brought about by long travel or active vacations. What better time to try the natural and sweet smelling remedy?

To travel with lavender, simply purchase ½ ounce (14g) of Bulgarian lavender essential oil from a reputable supplier, and place about ½ cup dried lavender buds into an airtight bag. Place both the bottle and the bag into your cosmetic case or carry-on bag, and you have instant portable first aid! For stale hotel rooms, place the dried buds into a shallow bowl, or even a cup from the mini bar, and leave in a central location of the room. Lavender oil can also be diffused into the room via a coffee filter.

Lavender Tea

The German version of the FDA is known as the Commision E. The Commision E posts monographs for herbs they approve of for medicinal use. Lavender flowers are approved for use as a tea in cases of insomnia, restlessness, and nervous stomach irritations. The sweet and mild taste of lavender tea, however, makes it hard to save and use only for these special occasions.

tea ball or bag
7 teaspoons lavender buds
4 teaspoons mint
honey (optional)

Place herbs in a tea ball or tea bag. Steep in a pot of boiling water (about 6 cups) for 4–6 minutes. Remove herbs and add honey to taste.

Muscle Rub

Sore muscles are often the remembrance of an adventure-filled weekend or a morning at the gym. You don't have to simply let the soreness run its course, however. Lavender rub not only provides much-needed relief, but its aroma is just the thing to transition your mind back to the days at hand. Use these blends as you would a massage oil and rub into sore muscles.

Essential Oil Version

¼ cup grapeseed oil
20 drops lavender oil

Blend together and pour into a 2-ounce (57g) bottle. Shake well and cap.

Dried Buds Version

1 cup grapeseed oil
½ cup dried lavender buds

Steep the flowers in the oil for 4–5 weeks. Strain the flowers and pour the oil into an 8-ounce bottle. Cap and use within 4 months.
Note: Lengthen the shelf life of oils by storing them in the fridge.

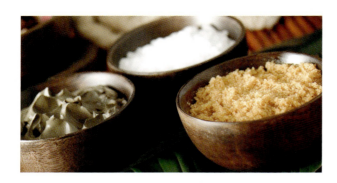

Invigorating Body Scrub

This body scrub is best used in the morning, as the scrubbing action and rejuvenating power of the lavender will be the lasting effects of this treatment.

2 cups sea salt
¼ cup grapeseed oil
30 drops lavender oil

Combine all ingredients thoroughly. Add more or less grapeseed oil to make the scrub the consistency you desire. (Remember, the oil is not water-soluble and will cause the shower to be slippery.) Scoop into a shallow jar and label with the ingredients and date.

To use: Scoop a small handful into your palm and scrub in a circular motion where desired. As you scrub, the salt will dissolve, and the oil will moisturize. Rinse well, then towel dry.

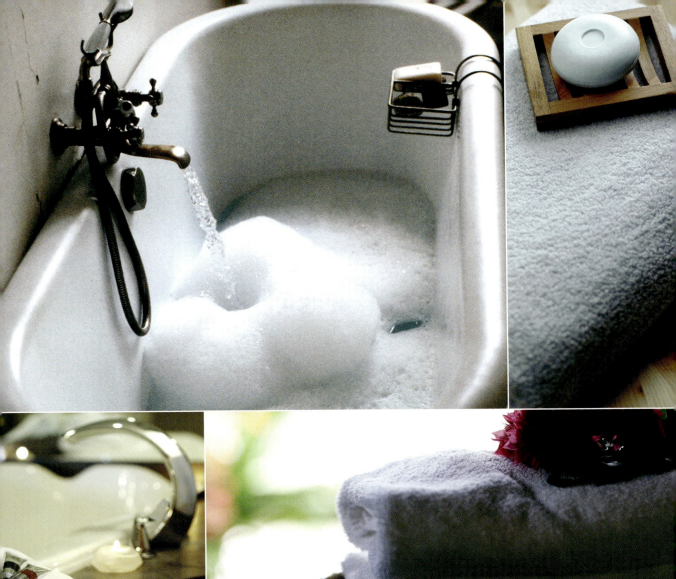

Crafts

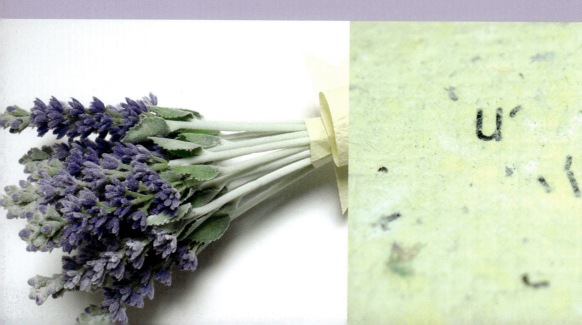

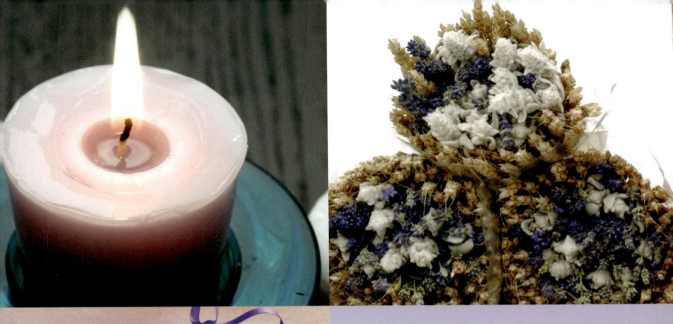

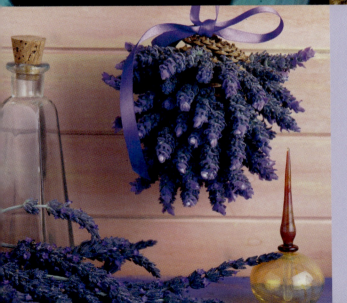

creation is a better means of *self-expression* than possession; it is through creating, not possessing, that life is *revealed.*

vida d. scudder

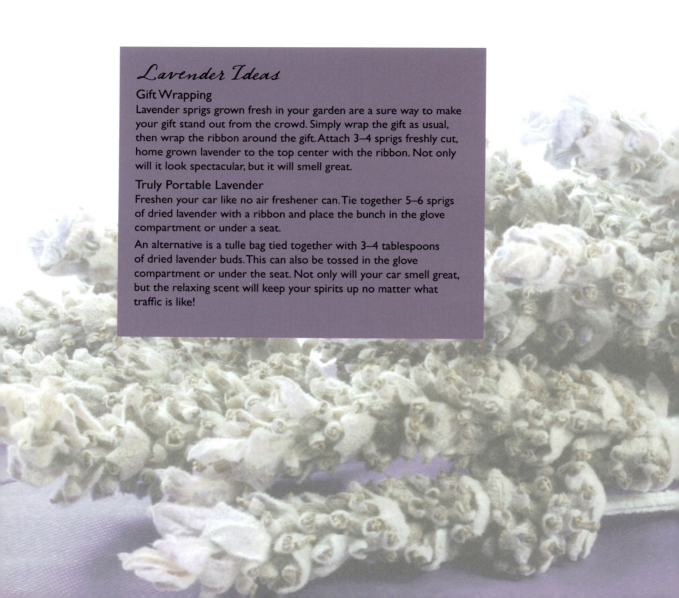

Lavender Ideas

Gift Wrapping

Lavender sprigs grown fresh in your garden are a sure way to make your gift stand out from the crowd. Simply wrap the gift as usual, then wrap the ribbon around the gift. Attach 3–4 sprigs freshly cut, home grown lavender to the top center with the ribbon. Not only will it look spectacular, but it will smell great.

Truly Portable Lavender

Freshen your car like no air freshener can. Tie together 5–6 sprigs of dried lavender with a ribbon and place the bunch in the glove compartment or under a seat.

An alternative is a tulle bag tied together with 3–4 tablespoons of dried lavender buds. This can also be tossed in the glove compartment or under the seat. Not only will your car smell great, but the relaxing scent will keep your spirits up no matter what traffic is like!

Lavender Sachets

Lavender sachets are the quintessential lavender craft. With numerous possibilities and uses, these little treats are certainly worth every bit of their reputation.

muslin drawstring bag
¼ cup dried lavender

Simply toss the lavender into the muslin bag, and pull the ends together and tie. These can be placed in a closet, drawer, behind sofa cushions, under the seat of the car, or anywhere a lavender fragrance is desired. The top can be sewn together to prevent leakage.

Lavender Candles

dried lavender stalks
white candle, 4 inches (10cm) in diameter, 6–8 inches (15–20 cm) tall
wire

Arrange the lavender around the candle so that the tops are an inch below the candle top. Cut the bottom of the stalks so they are flush with the bottom of the candle. Wrap the center with wire and secure. Wrap once more above and below for a total of three wire loops. Use caution when burning the candle, and trim the stalks if they get too close to the wax.

Heart Wreath

heart-shaped straw wreath support
dried lavender stalks
wire
lavender ribbon, 2 inches wide, 1 yard long

Arrange the stalks around the wreath, starting at the bottom point of the heart, with the flowering tops pointing towards the top. Begin with the bottom and wrap wire around the stalks just under the buds. Move upwards until all stalks are secured. With the ribbon, tie a small bow at the top, leaving the ends available to hang the wreath.

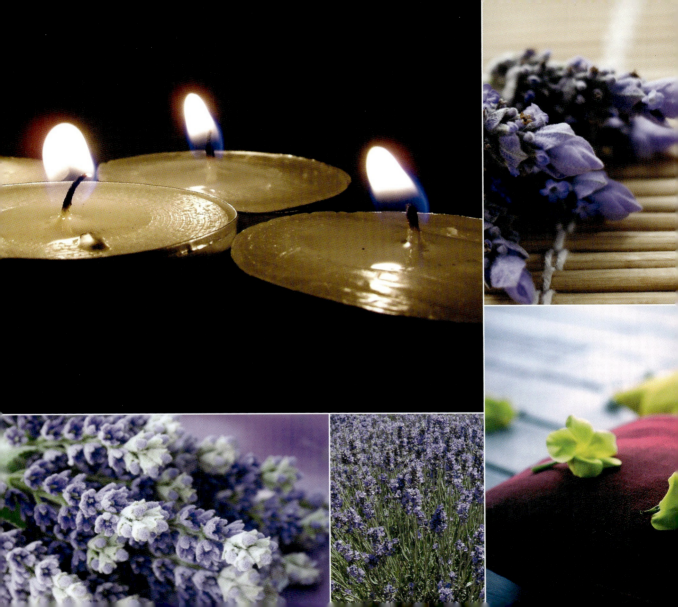

Handmade Lavender Paper

old towels
paper towels (must be plain white)
warm water
/½ cup dried lavender buds
paper mold (or make one with a fine mesh wire sheet framed with wood)

With an old towel or hand towel folded in half, make a soft place for the paper to dry. Set aside. Tear the paper towels into tiny sections. You will need 2 cups total. Add enough warm water to cover the paper (about ¾ cup). This is your pulp. Mix the pulp until there are no large clumps. Pour the pulp into a larger bowl and add about 1–2 cups water until the mixture resembles a thick soup. Now you have slurry. Add the ½ cup lavender to the slurry and be sure it is well incorporated. Take your screen and slide it into the slurry. Swish it around a little until it is well covered. Gently lift it out. It should be fully covered, with no thin spots. Allow to drip dry for a minute, then turn it out very gently onto the prepared towel to dry. It should take about a week to dry, depending on the humidity. When it is dry, just peel off and use as decorative cards, stationary, notes, etc.

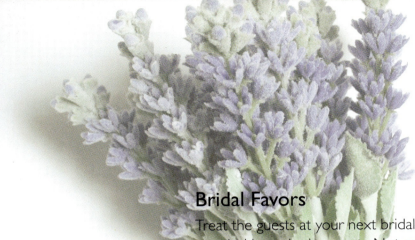

Bridal Favors

Treat the guests at your next bridal luncheon with lovely and practical lavender bouquets. Not only will the guests take home a party keepsake, but they will enjoy the scent for days afterwards. Be sure to make one for yourself as well!

purple cardstock 2x4 inches (5 x 10cm)
silver pen
purple ribbon (6–8 inches/ 15-20cm)
4–6 sprigs fresh lavender

Punch a hole in the corner of the cardstock, and with a silver pen, write the name of the guest. Using the ribbon, tie together the lavender and attach to the front of the card. Place in the center of the guest's plate on top of a purple napkin.

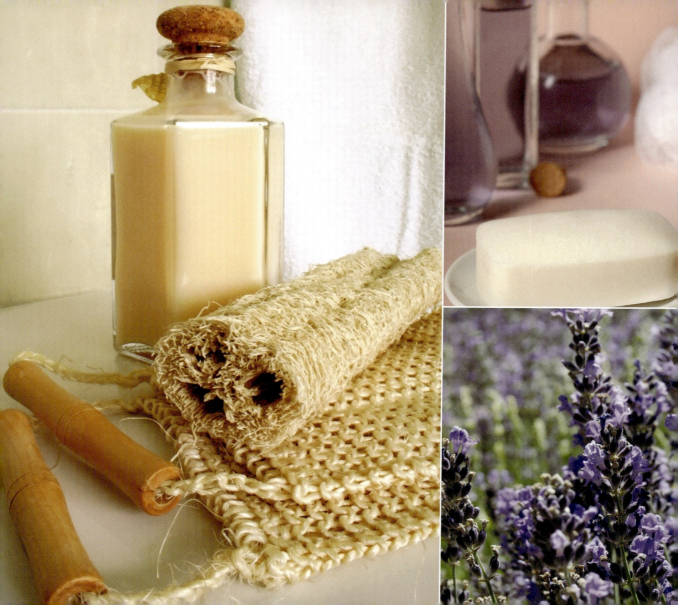

Milk and Lavender Bath

Enjoy lavender's relaxing fragrance while soothing your skin in this luxurious combo.

2 cups dried milk powder
¼ cup dried lavender buds
½ cup ground oats
25 drops lavender essential oil

Mix all ingredients well. Place in a blender or food processor and pulse to blend. If desired, pulse longer to break up the lavender buds. Place in an airtight jar and scoop ¼ cup into a warm bath.

Rolled Lavender Soaps

Lavender makes the perfect addition to any powder room or guest bath. Enhance your guests' stay with these easy-to-make, single-sized guest soaps.

2 cups dried lavender buds, separated
4 bars (or the equivalent in scraps—about 4.5 oz/128g) unscented soap
  (such as Ivory)
25 drops lavender essential oil

Place 1 cup of the buds in a shallow bowl, set aside. Grate the soap into fine bits. Add ½–1 cup warm water and place on the stove to melt the soap. "Cook" over low heat about 15 minutes until the soap and water are fully blended and the mixture resembles a thick pudding (it may have small chunks remaining). Add 1 cup of the lavender buds and the oil, and mix well. With clean dry hands, roll into balls, roughly 2–3 inches (5–7cm) in diameter, then roll through the lavender buds. Set on parchment paper to dry. Gently turn the soap daily until thoroughly dry. It should take about 3 or 4 days.

Lavender Bath Infusion

This luxurious treat is also fun for kids to add to their bath. Try adding one to your child's evening bath and let the lavender aroma ready your little one for a night full of sweet dreams.

1 cup baking soda
½ cup citric acid
½ cup sea salts
¼ cup cocoa butter, melted
2½ tablespoons grapeseed oil
¾ tablespoon liquid glycerin
25 drops lavender essential oil

Combine all the dry ingredients in a bowl. Mix well. Slowly add the cocoa butter, then the oils and glycerin. Blend until the mixture becomes the texture of cookie dough. Mold into small 2-inch balls and place on waxed paper to dry. As the cocoa butter cools, the lavender balls will harden. Let sit 24–48 hours, then store in a dry, airtight container.

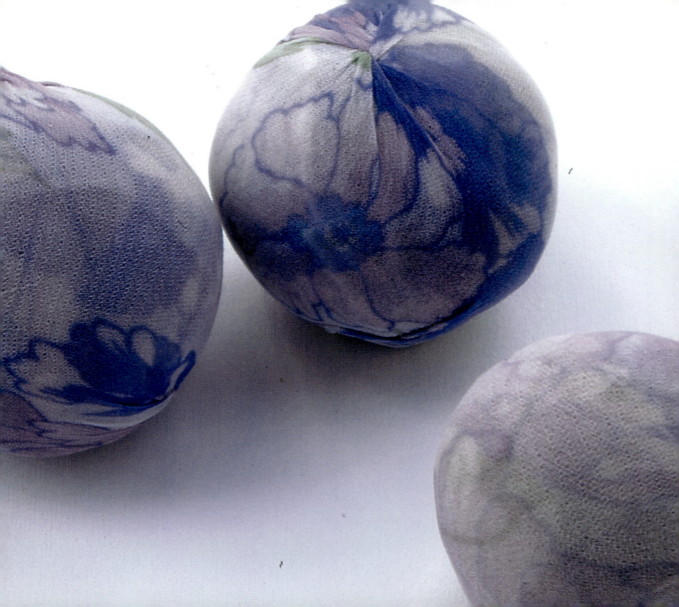

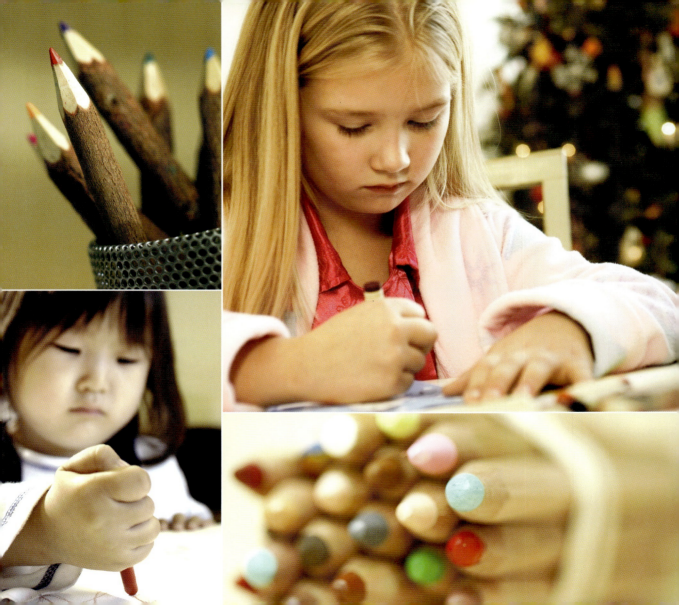

For Kids

Kids can help with many of the projects in this book, but the following especially offer a fun way for kids to enjoy lavender. Get creative—kids can take part in sprinkling lavender over their favorite sugar cookies, they can tie ribbons on your projects, or they can make their own, as shown below.

Greeting Cards

cardstock
glue stick
lavender flowers
envelopes

Have the child draw a person on the front of the card. Make sure they do not draw hair. With the glue, cover the entire spot over the head where the hair goes. Have the child sprinkle lavender buds in place of the hair on the person. Set aside to dry. Make several cards and use for Mother's day or for grandparents' birthdays.

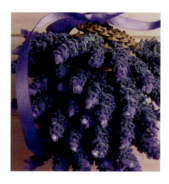

Lavender Ornaments

These lavender balls work great as holiday ornaments or springtime decorations. They also look good on gifts alongside the greeting card.

ribbon
toothpick
glue gun
Styrofoam balls
tack (optional)
+kid's craft glue
dried lavender buds

To prepare the craft, tie the ends of the ribbon making a big loop. With a toothpick and a dab of glue, poke the knotted end of the looped ribbon into the ball. (A tack may also be helpful in securing the ribbon in the Styrofoam ball.) Give the prepared ball to the child to cover with glue and lavender.